The
Essential Writings
of
Dr Edward Bach

The Essential Writings of Dr Edward Bach

The Twelve Healers and Other Remedies & Heal Thyself

Dr Edward Bach

MB, BS, DPH

With a preface by Judy Ramsell Howard SRN, SCM, HV

Custodian of the Bach Centre Heritage

Vermilion
LONDON

3 5 7 9 10 8 6 4 2

Copyright © Dr Edward Bach Centre 2005

The Twelve Healers and Other Remedies first published in Great Britain in
1933; new and revised edition 1934; new and enlarged edition 1936;
second enlarged edition 1941; reprinted 1946, 1949; reprinted with revisions
1952; reprinted 1955, 1960, 1964, 1968, 1971, 1973, 1974, 1975, 1977, 1979, 1983,
1986, 1988, 1989, 1990, 1991, 1993, 1994, 1996, 1997, 1999

Heal Thyself first published in Great Britain in 1931; reprinted 1937, 1946,
1949, 1953, 1957, 1962, 1966, 1970, 1973, 1974, 1976, 1978, 1979, 1981, 1984,
1985, 1986, 1987, 1988 (twice), 1989, 1990, 1991, 1992, 1993, 1994;
new edition 1996, 1997, 1999, 2003

All rights reserved. No part of this publication may be reproduced,
stored in a retrieval system, or transmitted in any form or by any means,
electronic, mechanical, photocopying, recording or otherwise,
without the prior permission of the copyright owner

This new edition first published in the UK in 2005 by Vermilion,
an imprint of Ebury Publishing, Random House,
20 Vauxhall Bridge Road, London SW1V 2SA

Random House Australia (Pty) Limited
20 Alfred Street, Milsons Point, Sydney,
New South Wales 2061, Australia

Random House New Zealand Limited
18 Poland Road, Glenfield,
Auckland 10, New Zealand

Random House (Pty) Limited
Isle of Houghton, Corner of Boundary Road & Carse O'Gowrie
Houghton 2198, South Africa

The Random House Group Limited Reg. No. 954009
www.randomhouse.co.uk

Papers used by Vermilion are natural, recyclable products
made from wood grown in sustainable forests.

Printed and bound in Great Britain by
Bookmarque Ltd, Croydon, Surrey

A CIP catalogue record for this book is available from the British Library

ISBN 9780091906726 (from Jan 2007)
ISBN 0091906725

Contents

PREFACE

Dr Edward Bach devoted his life to finding a simple and effective answer to people's distress. Through research and the rigorous study of human nature, he became convinced that at the heart of all distress and disease lay an imbalance in emotional outlook: our fear, suspicion, anger, greed, discouragement and other negative feelings may stand in the way of our contentment, joy, inner peace and good health.

Bach was a perfectionist and wanted to avoid confusion at all costs. This led him to destroy much of his work – papers, tinctures, active material and equipment were disposed of periodically. He said 'once a house is built, there is no need for the scaffolding', and, indeed, the complete 'house' was the series of thirty-eight Bach Flower Remedies that are now known and used throughout the world.

During his quest to discover the healing properties of the remedies, Dr Bach wasted no time in presenting his findings to the world. Having discovered twelve remedies he wrote *The Twelve Healers*. This was followed by *The Twelve Healers and Four Helpers*, and then *The Twelve Healers and Seven Helpers*. When he finally declared his work to be complete, he wrote the last text, *The Twelve Healers and Other Remedies*.

Throughout a period of some six years, Dr Bach considered the significance of his findings and questioned whether any link could be made between the remedies and astrology or other arts and sciences. Several theories have been expressed since as to whether there may be a numerological significance, or whether the order in which the remedies were discovered bore any relationship to Bach's own journey in life. There are several interesting suggestions and some that make valid and plausible conjecture. But whilst we may speculate all we like, we should also bear in mind the simplicity at the heart of all Dr Bach's work. Part of the simplicity lies in how Bach drew together his enormous discovery – the culmination of his life's work – into a simple text that everyone could read and use as a means of understanding how the remedies might help them. To this effect, in *The Twelve Healers and Other Remedies*, the reader is advised that 'they who will obtain the greatest benefit from this God-sent Gift will be those who keep it pure as it is; free from science, free from theories, for everything in Nature is simple'.

The thirty-eight Bach remedies are now well established and are becoming more and more accepted as a mainstream complementary therapy. But what lies behind them is a remarkable philosophy; a template to live by and aspire to. The remedies are very much part of achieving that philosophy – essentially, they are a means by which our individual potential may be reached.

Dr Bach set pen to paper and, on a cliff-top in North Wales, wrote *Heal Thyself*, his vision of the true meaning of health and disease. *Heal Thyself*, first published in 1931, and *The Twelve Healers and Other Remedies*, first published in 1933, were the only texts Bach did not attempt to destroy, and they have both remained in continuous print ever since.

The Essential Writings of Dr Edward Bach conveniently brings both booklets together in one volume, providing readers with the opportunity to appreciate the philosophy of Dr Edward Bach, and to develop a deeper understanding of how the thirty-eight Bach Flower Remedies can assist them in the process of self-healing as they find and explore their own pathway to health and inner freedom.

With best wishes

JUDY RAMSELL HOWARD
Custodian of the Bach Centre Heritage

The Twelve Healers and Other Remedies

This system of treatment is the most perfect which has been given to mankind within living memory. It has the power to cure disease; and, in its simplicity, it may be used in the household.

It is its simplicity, combined with its all-healing effects, that is so wonderful.

No science, no knowledge is necessary, apart from the simple methods described herein; and they who will obtain the greatest benefit from this God-sent Gift will be those who keep it pure as it is; free from science, free from theories, for everything in Nature is simple.

This system of healing, which has been Divinely revealed unto us, shows that it is our fears, our cares, our anxieties and such like that open the path to the invasion of illness. Thus by treating our fears, our cares, our worries and so on, we not only free ourselves from our illness, but the Herbs given unto us by the Grace of the Creator of all, in addition take away our fears and worries, and leave us happier and better in ourselves.

As the Herbs heal our fears, our anxieties, our worries, our faults and our failings, it is these we must seek, and then the disease, no matter what it is, will leave us.

There is little more to say, for the understanding mind will know all this, and may there be sufficient of those with understanding minds, unhampered by the trend of science, to use these Gifts of God for the relief and the blessing of those around them.

Thus, behind all disease lie our fears, our anxieties, our greed, our likes and dislikes. Let us seek these out and heal them, and with the healing of them will go the disease from which we suffer.

From time immemorial it has been known that Providential Means has placed in Nature the prevention and cure of disease, by means of divinely enriched herbs and plants and trees. The remedies of Nature given in this book have proved that they are blest above others in their work of mercy; and that they have been given the power to heal all types of illness and suffering.

In treating cases with these remedies no notice is taken of the nature of the disease. The individual is treated, and as he becomes well the disease goes, having been cast off by the increase of health.

All know that the same disease may have different effects on different people; it is the effects that need treatment, because they guide to the real cause.

The mind being the most delicate and sensitive part of the body, shows the onset and the course of disease much more definitely than the body, so that the outlook of mind is chosen as the guide as to which remedy or remedies are necessary.

In illness there is a change of mood from that in ordinary life, and those who are observant can notice this change often before, and sometimes long before, the disease appears, and by treatment can prevent the malady ever appearing. When illness has been present for some time, again the mood of the sufferer will guide to the correct remedy.

Take no notice of the disease, think only of the outlook on life of the one in distress.

Thirty-eight different states are simply described: and there should be no difficulty either for oneself, or for another, to find that state or a mixture of states which are present, and so to be able to give the required remedies to effect a cure.

The title, *The Twelve Healers,* has been retained for this book, as it is familiar to many readers.

The relief of suffering was so certain and beneficial, even when there were only twelve remedies, that it was deemed necessary to bring these before the attention of the public at the time, without waiting for the discovery of the remaining twenty-six, which complete the series. The original twelve are indicated by asterisks.

EDWARD BACH

THE 38 REMEDIES
are placed under the following
7 HEADINGS

THE 38 REMEDIES

For Those Who Have Fear

* Rock Rose

The remedy of emergency for cases where there even appears no hope. In accident or sudden illness, or when the patient is very frightened or terrified, or if the condition is serious enough to cause great fear to those around. If the patient is not conscious the lips may be moistened with the remedy. Other remedies in addition may also be required, as, for example, if there is unconsciousness, which is a deep, sleepy state, Clematis; if there is torture, Agrimony, and so on.

*Mimulus

Fear of worldly things, illness, pain, accidents, poverty, of dark, of being alone, of misfortune. The fears of everyday life. These people quietly and secretly bear their dread, they do not freely speak of it to others.

Cherry Plum

Fear of the mind being over-strained, of reason giving way, of doing fearful and dreaded things, not wished and known wrong, yet there comes the thought and impulse to do them.

ASPEN

Vague unknown fears, for which there can be given no explanation, no reason.

Yet the patient may be terrified of something terrible going to happen, he knows not what.

These vague unexplainable fears may haunt by night or day.

Sufferers are often afraid to tell their trouble to others.

RED CHESTNUT

For those who find it difficult not to be anxious for other people.

Often they have ceased to worry about themselves, but for those of whom they are fond they may suffer much, frequently anticipating that some unfortunate thing may happen to them.

For Those Who Suffer Uncertainty

*Cerato

Those who have not sufficient confidence in themselves to make their own decisions.

They constantly seek advice from others, and are often misguided.

*Scleranthus

Those who suffer much from being unable to decide between two things, first one seeming right then the other.

They are usually quiet people, and bear their difficulty alone, as they are not inclined to discuss it with others.

* Gentian

Those who are easily discouraged. They may be progressing well in illness or in the affairs of their daily life, but any small delay or hindrance to progress causes doubt and soon disheartens them.

Gorse

Very great hopelessness, they have given up belief that more can be done for them.

Under persuasion or to please others they may try different treatments, at the same time assuring those around that there is so little hope of relief.

HORNBEAM

For those who feel that they have not sufficient strength, mentally or physically, to carry the burden of life placed upon them; the affairs of every day seem too much for them to accomplish, though they generally succeed in fulfilling their task.

For those who believe that some part, of mind or body, needs to be strengthened before they can easily fulfil their work.

WILD OAT

Those who have ambitions to do something of prominence in life, who wish to have much experience, and to enjoy all that which is possible for them, to take life to the full.

Their difficulty is to determine what occupation to follow; as although their ambitions are strong, they have no calling which appeals to them above all others.

This may cause delay and dissatisfaction.

Not Sufficient Interest in Present Circumstances

* Clematis

Those who are dreamy, drowsy, not fully awake, no great interest in life. Quiet people, not really happy in their present circumstances, living more in the future than in the present; living in hopes of happier times, when their ideals may come true. In illness some make little or no effort to get well, and in certain cases may even look forward to death, in the hope of better times; or maybe, meeting again some beloved one whom they have lost.

Honeysuckle

Those who live much in the past, perhaps a time of great happiness, or memories of a lost friend, or ambitions which have not come true. They do not expect further happiness such as they have had.

Wild Rose

Those who without apparently sufficient reason become resigned to all that happens, and just glide through life, take it as it is, without any effort to improve things and find some joy.

They have surrendered to the struggle of life without complaint.

Olive

Those who have suffered much mentally or physically and are so exhausted and weary that they feel they have no more strength to make any effort. Daily life is hard work for them, without pleasure.

White Chestnut

For those who cannot prevent thoughts, ideas, arguments which they do not desire from entering their minds. Usually at such times when the interest of the moment is not strong enough to keep the mind full.

Thoughts which worry and will remain, or if for a time thrown out, will return. They seem to circle round and round and cause mental torture.

The presence of such unpleasant thoughts drives out peace and interferes with being able to think only of the work or pleasure of the day.

Mustard

Those who are liable to times of gloom, or even despair, as though a cold dark cloud overshadowed them and hid the light and the joy of life. It may not be possible to give any reason or explanation for such attacks.

Under these conditions it is almost impossible to appear happy or cheerful.

Chestnut Bud

For those who do not take full advantage of observation and experience, and who take a longer time than others to learn the lessons of daily life.

Whereas one experience would be enough for some, such people find it necessary to have more, sometimes several, before the lesson is learnt.

Therefore, to their regret, they find themselves having to make the same error on different occasions when once would have been enough, or observation of others could have spared them even that one fault.

LONELINESS

*WATER VIOLET

For those who in health or illness like to be alone. Very quiet people, who move about without noise, speak little, and then gently. Very independent, capable and self-reliant. Almost free of the opinions of others. They are aloof, leave people alone and go their own way. Often clever and talented. Their peace and calmness is a blessing to those around them.

*IMPATIENS

Those who are quick in thought and action and who wish all things to be done without hesitation or delay. When ill they are anxious for a hasty recovery.

They find it very difficult to be patient with people who are slow, as they consider it wrong and a waste of time, and they will endeavour to make such people quicker in all ways.

They often prefer to work and think alone, so that they can do everything at their own speed.

HEATHER

Those who are always seeking the companionship of anyone who may be available, as they find it necessary to discuss their own affairs with others, no matter whom it may be. They are very unhappy if they have to be alone for any length of time.

Over-Sensitive to Influences and Ideas

*Agrimony

The jovial, cheerful, humorous people who love peace and are distressed by argument or quarrel, to avoid which they will agree to give up much.

Though generally they have troubles and are tormented and restless and worried in mind or in body, they hide their cares behind their humour and jesting and are considered very good friends to know. They often take alcohol or drugs in excess, to stimulate themselves and help themselves bear their trials with cheerfulness.

*Centaury

Kind, quiet, gentle people who are over-anxious to serve others. They overtax their strength in their endeavours.

Their wish so grows upon them that they become more servants than willing helpers. Their good nature leads them to do more than their own share of work, and in so doing they may neglect their own particular mission in life.

WALNUT

For those who have definite ideals and ambitions in life and are fulfilling them, but on rare occasions are tempted to be led away from their own ideas, aims and work by the enthusiasm, convictions or strong opinions of others.

The remedy gives constancy and protection from outside influences.

HOLLY

For those who are sometimes attacked by thoughts of such kind as jealousy, envy, revenge, suspicion.

For the different forms of vexation.

Within themselves they may suffer much, often when there is no real cause for their unhappiness.

For Despondency or Despair

Larch

For those who do not consider themselves as good or capable as those around them, who expect failure, who feel that they will never be a success, and so do not venture or make a strong enough attempt to succeed.

Pine

For those who blame themselves. Even when successful they think they could have done better, and are never content with their efforts or the results. They are hard-working and suffer much from the faults they attach to themselves.

Sometimes if there is any mistake it is due to another, but they will claim responsibility even for that.

Elm

Those who are doing good work, are following the calling of their life and who hope to do something of importance, and this often for the benefit of humanity.

At times there may be periods of depression when they feel that the task they have undertaken is too difficult, and not within the power of a human being.

SWEET CHESTNUT

For those moments which happen to some people when the anguish is so great as to seem to be unbearable.

When the mind or body feels as if it had borne to the uttermost limit of its endurance, and that now it must give way.

When it seems there is nothing but destruction and annihilation left to face.

STAR OF BETHLEHEM

For those in great distress under conditions which for a time produce great unhappiness.

The shock of serious news, the loss of someone dear, the fright following an accident, and such like.

For those who for a time refuse to be consoled, this remedy brings comfort.

WILLOW

For those who have suffered adversity or misfortune and find these difficult to accept, without complaint or resentment, as they judge life much by the success which it brings.

They feel that they have not deserved so great a trial, that it was unjust, and they become embittered.

They often take less interest and are less active in those things of life which they had previously enjoyed.

OAK

For those who are struggling and fighting strongly to get well, or in connection with the affairs of their daily life. They will go on trying one thing after another, though their case may seem hopeless.

They will fight on. They are discontented with themselves if illness interferes with their duties or helping others.

They are brave people, fighting against great difficulties, without loss of hope or effort.

CRAB APPLE

This is the remedy of cleansing.

For those who feel as if they had something not quite clean about themselves.

Often it is something of apparently little importance: in others there may be more serious disease which is almost disregarded compared to the one thing on which they concentrate.

In both types they are anxious to be free from the one particular thing which is greatest in their minds and which seems so essential to them that it should be cured.

They become despondent if treatment fails.

Being a cleanser, this remedy purifies wounds if the patient has reason to believe that some poison has entered which must be drawn out.

Over-Care for Welfare of Others

*Chicory

Those who are very mindful of the needs of others they tend to be over-full of care for children, relatives, friends, always finding something that should be put right. They are continually correcting what they consider wrong, and enjoy doing so. They desire that those for whom they care should be near them.

*Vervain

Those with fixed principles and ideas, which they are confident are right, and which they very rarely change.

They have a great wish to convert all around them to their own views of life.

They are strong of will and have much courage when they are convinced of those things that they wish to teach.

In illness they struggle on long after many would have given up their duties.

Vine

Very capable people, certain of their own ability, confident of success.

Being so assured, they think that it would be for the benefit of others if they could be persuaded to do things as they themselves do, or as they are certain is right. Even in illness they will direct their attendants.

They may be of great value in emergency.

BEECH

For those who feel the need to see more good and beauty in all that surrounds them. And, although much appears to be wrong, to have the ability to see the good growing within. So as to be able to be more tolerant, lenient and understanding of the different way each individual and all things are working to their own final perfection.

ROCK WATER

Those who are very strict in their way of living; they deny themselves many of the joys and pleasures of life because they consider it might interfere with their work.

They are hard masters to themselves. They wish to be well and strong and active, and will do anything which they believe will keep them so. They hope to be examples which will appeal to others who may then follow their ideas and be better as a result.

The English and botanical name of each
remedy is as follows:

AGRIMONY	*Agrimonia eupatoria*
ASPEN	*Populus tremula*
BEECH	*Fagus sylvatica*
CENTAURY	*Centaurium umbellatum*
CERATO	*Ceratostigma willmottiana*
CHERRY PLUM	*Prunus cerasifera*
CHESTNUT BUD	*AEsculus hippocastanum*
CHICORY	*Cichorium intybus*
CLEMATIS	*Clematis vitalba*
CRAB APPLE	*Malus pumila*
ELM	*Ulmus procera*
GENTIAN	*Gentiana amarella*
GORSE	*Ulex europoeus*
HEATHER	*Calluna vulgaris*
HOLLY	*Ilex aquifolium*
HONEYSUCKLE	*Lonicera caprifolium*
HORNBEAM	*Carpinus betulus*
IMPATIENS	*Impatiens glandulifera*
LARCH	*Larix decidua*
MIMULUS	*Mimulus guttatus*
MUSTARD	*Sinapis arvensis*
OAK	*Quercus robur*
OLIVE	*Olea europoea*

PINE	*Pinus sylvestris*
RED CHESTNUT	*AEsculus carnea*
ROCK ROSE	*Helianthemum nummularium*
ROCK WATER	*Aqua Petra*
SCLERANTHUS	*Scleranthus annuus*
STAR OF BETHLEHEM	*Ornithogalum umbetelatum*
SWEET CHESTNUT	*Castanea sativa*
VERVAIN	*Verbena officinalis*
VINE	*Vitis vinifera*
WALNUT	*Juglans regia*
WATER VIOLET	*Hottonia palustris*
WHITE CHESTNUT	*AEsculus hippocastanum*
WILD OAT	*Bromus ramosus†*
WILD ROSE	*Rosa canina*
WILLOW	*Salix vitellina*

†There is no English name for Bromus ramosus. Bromus is an ancient word meaning Oat. (The alteration in the Latin names of certain of the plants in this edition of *The Twelve Healers* is due to changes of nomenclature governed by The International Rules of Botanical Nomenclature.)

THE COMPOSITE RESCUE REMEDY

Dr Bach combined five specific Remedies from the 38 to formulate an emergency composite that he chose to call 'Rescue Remedy'. He saved a fisherman's life in 1930 with this preparation.

Its purpose is to treat the pre or post emotional effect that a sufferer may experience through shock, great fear or terror, panic, severe mental stress and tension, a feeling of desperation or a numbed, bemused state of mind.

To nullify the sufferer's shock and fear is of the utmost importance in helping the natural healing process of one's being to proceed without hindrance. Shock, terror and panic can manifest in minor traumas as well as in the more serious states of emergency. A brief definition of 'emergency' would be e.g. when in mental or physical shock, terror and panic, various emotional upsets (bereavement, stage fright, visiting the dentist, general nervous debility, trauma etc.). Even severe bites and stings create the effects of shock and panic.

Rescue Remedy can be taken along with any of the other 38 Remedies if required - please see general instructions (see page 31), also for reference to the **Rescue Remedy Cream** preparation.

Note: It has to be remembered that each of the 5 remedies used in this composite can be equally efficient when taken as a separate entity as and when required.

Treatment of Animals

One can sometimes assess a particular personality trait or definite temperamental attitude in animals (viz. aggressiveness, possessiveness, lethargy, timidity, jealous etc.) and so they, as with humans, can be treated accordingly with one or more of the 38 remedies. The Rescue Remedy, although not being considered a panacea for all ills as far as humans are concerned, does act as an excellent all purpose basic remedy for animals, who react very favourably to this remedy irrespective of the state or cause of suffering.

Dosage: 4 drops of the Rescue Remedy stock concentrate (plus 2 drops from any other chosen remedy) in the animal's drink. A dilution can also be sprinkled over its food. For larger creatures needing to drink out of a bucket, the dosage would be in proportion to approximately 10 drops per gallon. 4 drops on a cube of sugar might be appropriate with some animals.

Methods of Dosage

The stock concentrates will keep indefinitely. They can be taken by people of all ages - there is no danger of an over-dose or side effects, and should the wrong choice be made no harm will ensue. They will not be influenced by, nor will they affect any form of medicine prescribed to a person.

Animals and plants also benefit from this treatment.

First determine the personality and temperament; fears, worries, emotional upsets and the subsequent effect in outlook and attitude. More than one remedy can be taken at the one time, but it should not be difficult to limit your choice to within six.

Dosage: Take 2 drops from each chosen stock remedy in a cup of water, fruit juice, or any beverage, and sip fairly frequently. Replenish cup to continue treatment if need be . . . ALTERNATIVELY you can put the drops in a bottle of approx. 1 fl.oz. (30ml) capacity and fill up with Natural Spring Water (non-gas) and take 4 drops on the tongue directly from the bottle. Take as often as needed but at least 4 times a day, especially first and last thing daily.

Hold the dose a moment or so in the mouth before swallowing to gain the full effect (this also applies when sipped from a cup). Such a prepared dosage bottle will remain fresh for about 3 weeks if stored in a cool place (fridge in very warm climates), but should a preservative be necessary, include a spoonful of brandy or cider vinegar to the preparation. Dosage drops can be added to a baby's bottle or taken in a spoonful of water.

Rescue Remedy can be included along with the others when needed, but use 4 drops instead of two as indicated for other remedies, and also count it as a single stock remedy rather than the five from which it is composed. When required for immediate or emergency use as a separate remedy take 4 drops in a cup of water and sip at intervals. If the sufferer is unable to swallow, or in a comatose state, then the lips, behind the ears and the wrists should be moistened with the Remedy. **It does not take the place of medical attention.**

External Application. For burns, scalds, stings, sprains etc. - apply a couple of drops direct from the Rescue Remedy stock bottle immediately to the affected area.

There is also available **Rescue Remedy Cream** which has been used for ulcers, lacerations, burns, scalds, sprains, massage and many other needs.

Note: If liquid is totally unavailable, then drops *can* be taken from the stock concentrate, but it must be emphasised for the benefit of abstainers, that this would mean a direct intake of brandy.

And may we ever have joy and gratitude in our hearts that the Great Creator of all things, in His Love for us, has placed the herbs in the fields for our healing.

Heal Thyself

An explanation of the real cause and cure of disease

This book is dedicated to
all who suffer or who are in distress

Foreword

Dr Bach is well known for his genuine mix of humble spirituality and down-to-earth understanding, and his simple philosophy has been a source of great inspiration and comfort to many people. *Heal Thyself* has aroused much interest which in turn has prompted certain questions about particular aspects of the book.

In the final paragraph we are urged to unite with 'that great band of the White Brotherhood'. Some people have expressed concern that this was a racist remark. We would like to make it absolutely clear that the use of the term had nothing whatsoever to do with skin colour or race or religion. In fact, Dr Bach found every form of racism abhorrent. Quite simply, he used the word 'white' to mean something light, bright, clean and fresh in origin, and he regarded everyone of like mind as being part of a common band or 'brotherhood'.

In Chapter 3 Dr Bach directly links physical symptoms to negative emotions. However, it is important to note that he wrote *Heal Thyself* at the very beginning of his discoveries. He later abandoned the idea that physical afflictions were a guide to underlying emotions, as clearly expressed in *The Twelve Healers and Other Remedies*: 'The mind being the most delicate and sensitive part of the body, shows the onset and the course of disease much more definitely than the body, so that the outlook of mind is chosen as the guide as to which remedy or remedies are necessary. Take no notice of the disease, think only of the outlook on life of the one in distress.'

We hope this has helped allay any misunderstanding, but most of all, we hope you enjoy the book and find your thoughts and perspective on life enriched as a result.

Happy reading and best wishes,

The Bach Centre, Mount Vernon

Chapter One

It is not the object of this book to suggest that the art of healing is unnecessary; far be from it any such intention; but it is humbly hoped that it will be a guide to those who suffer to seek within themselves the real origin of their maladies, so that they may assist themselves in their own healing. Moreover, it is hoped that it may stimulate those, both in the medical profession and in religious orders, who have the welfare of humanity at heart, to redouble their efforts in seeking the relief of human suffering, and so hasten that day when the victory over disease will be complete.

The main reason for the failure of modern medical science is that it is dealing with results and not causes. For many centuries the real nature of disease has been masked by materialism, and thus disease itself has been given every opportunity of extending its ravages, since it has not been attacked at its origin. The situation is like to an enemy strongly fortified in the hills, continually waging guerilla warfare in the country around, while the people, ignoring the fortified garrison, content themselves with repairing the damaged houses and burying the dead, which are the result of the raids of the marauders. So, generally speaking, is the situation in medicine to-day; nothing more than the patching up of those attacked and the burying of those who are slain, without a thought being given to the real stronghold.

Disease will never be cured or eradicated by present materialistic methods, for the simple reason that disease in its origin is not material. What we know as disease is an ultimate result produced in the body, the end product of deep and long acting forces, and even if material treatment alone is apparently successful this is nothing more than a temporary relief unless the real cause has been removed. The modern trend of medical science, by misinterpreting the true nature of disease and concentrating it in materialistic terms in the physical body, has enormously increased its power, firstly, by distracting the thoughts of people from its true origin and hence from the effective method of attack, and secondly, by localising it in the body, thus obscuring true hope of recovery and raising a mighty disease complex of fear, which never should have existed.

Disease is in essence the result of conflict between Soul and Mind, and will never be eradicated except by spiritual and mental effort. Such efforts, if properly made with understanding as we shall see later, can cure and prevent disease by removing those basic factors which are its primary cause. No effort directed to the body alone can do more than superficially repair damage, and in this there is no cure, since the cause is still operative and may at any moment again demonstrate its presence in another form. In fact, in many cases apparent recovery is harmful, since it hides from the patient the true cause of his trouble, and in the satisfaction of apparently renewed health the real factor, being unnoticed, may gain in strength. Contrast these cases with that of the patient who knows, or who is by some wise physician instructed in, the nature of the adverse spiritual or mental forces at work, the result of which has precipitated what we call disease in the physical body. If that patient directly attempts to neutralise those forces, health improves as soon as this is successfully begun, and when it is completed the disease will disappear. This is true healing by attacking the stronghold, the very base of the cause of suffering.

One of the exceptions to materialistic methods in modern science is that of the great Hahnemann, the founder of Homeopathy, who with his realisation of the beneficent love of the Creator and of the Divinity which resides within man, by studying the mental attitude of his patients towards life, environment and their respective diseases, sought to find in the herbs of the field and in the realms of nature the remedy which would not only heal their bodies but would at the same time uplift their mental outlook. May his science be extended and developed by those true physicians who have the love of humanity at heart.

Five hundred years before Christ some physicians of ancient India, working under the influence of the Lord Buddha, advanced the art of healing to so perfect a state that they were able to abolish surgery, although the surgery of their time was as efficient, or more so, than that of the present day. Such men as Hippocrates with his mighty ideals of healing, Paracelsus with his certainty of the divinity in man, and Hahnemann who realised that disease originated in a plane above the physical - all these knew much of the real nature and remedy of suffering. What untold misery would have been spared during the last twenty or twenty-five centuries had the teaching of these great masters of their art been followed, but, as in other things, materialism has appealed too strongly to the Western world, and for so long a time, that the voices of the practical obstructors have risen above the advice of those who knew the truth.

Let it be briefly stated that disease, though apparently so cruel, is in itself beneficent and for our good and, if rightly interpreted, it will guide us to our essential faults. If properly treated it will be the cause of the removal of those faults and leave us better and greater than before. Suffering is a corrective to point out a lesson which by other means we have failed to grasp, and never can it be eradicated until that lesson is learnt. Let it also be known that in those who understand and are able to read the significance of premonitory symptoms disease may be prevented before its onset or aborted in its earlier stages if the proper corrective spiritual and mental efforts be undertaken. Nor need any case despair, however severe, for the fact that the individual is still granted physical life indicates that the Soul who rules is not without hope.

CHAPTER TWO

To understand the nature of disease certain fundamental truths have to be acknowledged.

The first of these is that man has a Soul which is his real self; a Divine, Mighty Being, a Son of the Creator of all things, of which the body, although the earthly temple of that Soul, is but the minutest reflection: that our Soul, our Divinity Who resides in and around us, lays down for us our lives as He wishes them to be ordered and, so far as we will allow, ever guides, protects and encourages us, watchful and beneficent to lead us always for our utmost advantage: that He, our Higher Self, being a spark of the Almighty, is thereby invincible and immortal.

The second principle is that we, as we know ourselves in this world, are personalities down here for the purpose of gaining all the knowledge and experience which can be obtained through earthly existence, of developing virtues which we lack and of wiping out all that is wrong within us, thus advancing towards the perfection of our natures. The Soul knows what environment and what circumstances will best enable us to do this, and hence He places us in that branch of life most suited for that object.

Thirdly, we must realise that the short passage on this earth, which we know as life, is but a moment in the course of our evolution, as one day at school is to a life, and although we can for the present only see and comprehend that one day, our intuition tells us that birth was infinitely far from our beginning and death infinitely far from our ending. Our Souls, which are really we, are immortal, and the bodies of which we are conscious are temporary, merely as horses we ride to go a journey, or instruments we use to do a piece of work.

Then follows a fourth great principle, that so long as our Souls and personalities are in harmony all is joy and peace, happiness and health. It is when our personalities are led astray from the path laid down by the Soul, either by our own worldly desires or by the persuasion of others, that a conflict arises. This conflict is the root cause of disease and unhappiness. No matter what our work in the world – bootblack or monarch, landlord or peasant, rich or poor – so long as we do that particular work according to the dictates of the Soul, all is well; and we can further rest assured that in whatever station of life we are placed, princely or lowly, it contains the lessons and experiences necessary at the moment for our evolution, and gives us the best advantage for the development of ourselves.

The next great principle is the understanding of the Unity of all things: that the Creator of all things is Love, and that everything of which we are conscious is in all its infinite number of forms a manifestation of that Love, whether it be a planet or a pebble, a star or a dewdrop, man or the lowliest form of life. It may be possible to get a glimpse of this conception by thinking of our Creator as a great blazing sun of beneficence and love and from the centre an infinite number of beams radiate in every direction, and that we and all of which we are conscious are particles at the end of those beams, sent out to gain experience and knowledge, but ultimately to return to the great centre. And though to us each ray may appear separate and distinct, it is in reality part of the great central Sun. Separation is impossible, for as soon as a beam of light is cut off from its source it ceases to exist. Thus we may comprehend a little of the impossibility of separateness, as although each ray may have its individuality, it is nevertheless part of the great central creative power. Thus any action against ourselves or against another affects the whole, because by causing imperfection in a part it reflects on the whole, every particle of which must ultimately become perfect.

So we see there are two great possible fundamental errors: dissociation between our Souls and our personalities, and cruelty or wrong to others, for this is a sin against Unity. Either of these brings conflict, which leads to disease. An understanding of where we are making an error (which is so often not realised by us) and an earnest endeavour to correct the fault will lead not only to a life of joy and peace, but also to health.

Disease is in itself beneficent, and has for its object the bringing back of the personality to the Divine will of the Soul; and thus we can see that it is both preventable and avoidable, since if we could only realise for ourselves the mistakes we are making and correct these by spiritual and mental means there could be no need for the severe lessons of suffering. Every opportunity is given us by the Divine Power to mend our ways before, as a last resort, pain and suffering have to be applied. It may not be the errors of this life, this day at school, which we are combating; and although we in our physical minds may not be conscious of the reason of our suffering, which may to us appear cruel and without reason, yet our Souls (which are ourselves) know the full purpose and are guiding us to our best advantage. Nevertheless, understanding and correction of our errors would shorten our illness and bring us back to health. Knowledge of the Soul's purpose and acquiescence in that knowledge means the relief of earthly suffering and distress, and leaves us free to develop our evolution in joy and happiness.

There are two great errors: first, to fail to honour and obey the dictates of our Soul, and second, to act against Unity. On account of the former, be ever reluctant to judge others, because what is right for one is wrong for another. The merchant, whose work it is to build up a big trade not only to his own advantage but also to that of all those whom he may employ, thereby gaining knowledge of efficiency and control and developing the virtues associated with each, must of necessity use different qualities and different virtues from those of a nurse, sacrificing her life in the care of the sick; and yet both, if obeying the dictates of their Souls, are rightly learning those qualities necessary for their evolution. It is obeying the commands of our Soul, our Higher Self, which we learn through conscience, instinct and intuition, that matters.

Thus we see that by its very principles and in its very essence, disease is both preventable and curable, and it is the work of spiritual healers and physicians to give, in addition to material remedies, the knowledge to the suffering of the error of their lives, and of the manner in which these errors can be eradicated, and so to lead the sick back to health and joy.

CHAPTER THREE

What we know as disease is the terminal stage of a much deeper disorder, and to ensure complete success in treatment it is obvious that dealing with the final result alone will not be wholly effective unless the basic cause is also removed. There is one primary error which man can make, and that is action against Unity; this originates in self-love. So also we may say that there is but one primary affliction – discomfort, or disease. And as action against Unity may be divided into various types, so also may disease – the result of these actions – be separated into main groups corresponding to their causes. The very nature of an illness will be a useful guide to assist in discovering the type of action which is being taken against the Divine Law of Love and Unity.

If we have in our nature sufficient love of all things, then we can do no harm; because that love would stay our hand at any action, our mind at any thought which might hurt another. But we have not yet reached that state of perfection; if we had, there would be no need for our existence here. But all of us are seeking and advancing towards that state, and those of us who suffer in mind or body are by this very suffering being led towards that ideal condition; and if we will but read it aright, we may not only hasten our steps towards that goal, but also save ourselves illness and distress. From the moment the lesson is understood and the error eliminated there is no longer need for the correction, because we must remember that suffering is in itself beneficent, in that it points out to us when we are taking wrong paths and hastens our evolution to its glorious perfection.

The real primary diseases of man are such defects as pride, cruelty, hate, self-love, ignorance, instability and greed; and each of these, if considered, will be found to be adverse to Unity. Such defects as these are the real diseases (using the word in the modern sense), and it is a continuation and persistence in such defects after we have reached that stage of development when we know them to be wrong, which precipitates in the body the injurious results which we know as illness.

Pride is due, firstly, to lack of recognition of the smallness of the personality and its utter dependence on the Soul, and that all the successes it may have are not of itself but are blessings bestowed by the Divinity within; secondly, the loss of the sense of proportion, of the minuteness of one amidst the scheme of Creation. As Pride invariably refuses to bend with humility and resignation to the Will of the Great Creator, it commits actions contrary to that Will.

Cruelty is a denial of the unity of all and a failure to understand that any action adverse to another is in opposition to the whole, and hence an action against Unity. No man would practise its injurious effects against those near and dear to him, and by the law of Unity we have to grow until we understand that everyone, as being part of a whole, must become near and dear to us, until even those who persecute us call up only feelings of love and sympathy.

Hate is the opposite of Love, the reverse of the Law of Creation. It is contrary to the whole Divine scheme and is a denial of the Creator; it leads only to such actions and thoughts which are adverse to Unity and the opposite of those which would be dictated by Love.

Self-love again is a denial of Unity and the duty we owe to our brother men by putting the interests of ourselves before the good of humanity and the care and protection of those immediately around us.

Ignorance is the failure to learn, the refusal to see Truth when the opportunity is offered, and leads to many wrong acts such as can only exist in darkness and are not possible when the light of Truth and Knowledge is around us.

Instability, indecision and weakness of purpose result when the personality refuses to be ruled by the Higher Self, and lead us to betray others through our weakness. Such a condition would not be possible had we within us the knowledge of the Unconquerable Invincible Divinity which is in reality ourselves.

Greed leads to a desire for power. It is a denial of the freedom and individuality of every soul. Instead of recognising that every one of us is down here to develop freely upon his own lines according to the dictates of the soul alone, to increase his individuality, and to work free and unhampered, the personality with greed desires to dictate, mould and command, usurping the power of the Creator.

Such are examples of real disease, the origin and basis of all our suffering and distress. Each of such defects, if persisted in against the voice of the Higher Self, will produce a conflict which must of necessity be reflected in the physical body, producing its own specific type of malady.

We can now see how any type of illness from which we may suffer will guide us to the discovery of the fault which lies behind our affliction. For example, Pride, which is arrogance and rigidity of mind, will give rise to those diseases which produce rigidity and stiffness of the body. Pain is the result of cruelty, whereby the patient learns through personal suffering not to inflict it upon others, either from a physical or from a mental standpoint. The penalties of Hate are loneliness, violent uncontrollable temper, mental nerve storms and conditions of hysteria. The diseases of introspection – neurosis, neurasthenia and similar conditions – which rob life of so much enjoyment, are caused by excessive Self-love. Ignorance and lack of wisdom bring their own difficulties in everyday life, and in addition should there be a persistence in refusing to see truth when the opportunity has been given, short-sightedness and impairment of vision and hearing are the natural consequences. Instability of mind must lead to the same quality in the body with those various disorders which affect movement and co-ordination. The result of greed and domination of others is such diseases as will render the sufferer a slave to his own body, with desires and ambitions curbed by the malady.

Moreover, the very part of the body affected is no accident, but is in accordance with the law of cause and effect, and again will be a guide to help us. For example, the heart, the fountain of life and hence of love, is attacked when especially the love side of the nature towards humanity is not developed or is wrongly used; a hand affected denotes failure or wrong in action; the brain being the centre of control, if afflicted, indicates lack of control in the personality. Such must follow as the law lays down. We are all ready to admit the many results which may follow a fit of violent temper, the shock of sudden bad news; if trivial affairs can thus affect the body, how much more serious and deep-rooted must be a prolonged conflict between soul and body. Can we wonder that the result gives rise to such grievous complaints as the diseases amongst us to-day?

But yet there is no cause for depression. The prevention and cure of disease can be found by discovering the wrong within ourselves and eradicating this fault by the earnest development of the virtue which will destroy it; not by fighting the wrong, but by bringing in such a flood of its opposing virtue that it will be swept from our natures.

CHAPTER FOUR

So we find that there is nothing of the nature of accident as regards disease, either in its type or in that part of the body which is affected; like all other results of energy, it follows the law of cause and effect. Certain maladies may be caused by direct physical means, such as those associated with some poisons, accidents and injuries, and gross excesses; but disease in general is due to some basic error in our constitution, as in the examples already given.

And thus for a complete cure not only must physical means be used, choosing always the best methods which are known to the art of healing, but we ourselves must also endeavour to the utmost of our ability to remove any fault in our nature; because final and complete healing ultimately comes from within, from the Soul itself, which by His beneficence radiates harmony throughout the personality, when allowed to do so.

As there is one great root cause of all disease, namely self-love, so there is one great certain method of relief of all suffering, the conversion of self-love into devotion to others. If we but sufficiently develop the quality of losing ourselves in the love and care of those around us, enjoying the glorious adventure of gaining knowledge and helping others, our personal griefs and sufferings rapidly come to an end. It is the great ultimate aim: the losing of our own interests in the service of humanity. It matters not the station in life in which our Divinity has placed us. Whether engaged in trade or profession, rich or poor, monarch or beggar, for one and all it is possible to carry on the work of their respective vocations and yet be veritable blessings to those around by communicating to them the Divine Love of Brotherhood.

But the vast majority of us have some way to travel before we can reach this state of perfection, although it is surprising how rapidly any individual may advance along these lines if the effort is seriously made, providing he trusts not in his poor personality alone but has implicit faith, that by the example and teaching of the great masters of the world he may be enabled to unite himself with his own Soul, the Divinity within, when all things become possible. In most of us there is one, or more, adverse defect which is particularly hindering our advancement, and it is such defect, or defects, which we must especially seek out within ourselves, and whilst striving to develop and extend the love side of our nature towards the world, endeavour at the same time to wash away any such defect in particular by the flooding of our nature with the opposing virtue. At first this may be a little difficult, but only just at first, for it is remarkable how rapidly a truly encouraged virtue will increase, linked with the knowledge that with the aid of the Divinity within us, if we but persevere, failure is impossible.

In the development of Universal Love within ourselves we must learn to realise more and more that every human being, however lowly, is a son of the Creator, and that one day and in due time he will advance to perfection just as we all hope to do. However base a man or creature may appear, we must remember that there is the Divine Spark within, which will slowly but surely grow until the glory of the Creator irradiates that being.

Moreover, the question of right or wrong, of good and evil, is purely relative. That which is right in the natural evolution of the aboriginal would be wrong for the more enlightened of our civilisation, and that which might even be a virtue in such as ourselves might be out of place, and hence wrong, in one who has reached the stage of discipleship. What we call wrong or evil is in reality good out of place, and hence is purely relative. Let us remember also that our standard of idealism again is relative; to the animals we must appear as veritable gods, whereas we in ourselves are very far below the standards of the great White Brotherhood of Saints and Martyrs who have given their all to be examples to us. Hence we must have compassion and sympathy for the lowliest, for whilst we may consider ourselves as having advanced far above their level, we are in ourselves minute indeed, and have yet a long journey before us to reach the standard of our older brothers, whose light shines throughout the world in every age.

If Pride assails us, let us try to realise that our personalities are in themselves as nothing, unable to do any good work or acceptable service, or to resist the powers of darkness, unless assisted by that Light which is from above, the Light of our Soul; endeavour to comprehend a glimpse of the omnipotence and unthinkable mightiness of our Creator, Who makes in all perfection a world in one drop of water and systems upon systems of universes, and try to realise the relative humility we owe and our utter dependence upon Him. We learn to pay homage and give respect to our human superiors; how infinitely more should we acknowledge our own frailty with utmost humility before the Great Architect of the Universe!

If Cruelty, or Hate, bar our way to progress, let us remember that Love is the foundation of Creation, that in every living soul there is some good, and that in the best of us there is some bad. By seeking the good in others, even in those who at first offend us, we shall learn to develop, if nothing more, some sympathy and a hope that they will see better ways; then it follows that the desire will arise to help them to that uplift. The ultimate conquest of all will be through love and gentleness, and when we have sufficiently developed these two qualities nothing will be able to assail us, since we shall ever have compassion and not offer resistance; for, again, by the same law of cause and effect it is resistance which damages. Our object in life is to follow the dictates of our Higher Self, undeterred by the influence of others, and this can only be achieved if we gently go our own way, but at the same time never interfere with the personality of another or cause the least harm by any method of cruelty or hate. We must strive to learn love of others, beginning perhaps with one individual or even an animal, and let this love develop and extend over a wider and wider range, until its opposing defects will automatically disappear. Love begets Love, as Hate does Hate.

The cure of self-love is effected by the turning outwards to others of the care and attention which we are devoting to ourselves, becoming so engrossed in their welfare that we forget ourselves in that endeavour. As one great order of Brotherhood expresses it, 'to seek the solace of our own distress by extending relief and consolation to our fellow-creatures in the hour of their affliction,' and there is no surer way of curing self-love and the disorders which follow it than by such a method.

Instability can be eradicated by the development of self-determination, by making up the mind and doing things with definiteness instead of wavering and hovering. Even if at first we may sometimes make errors, it were better to act than to let opportunities pass for the want of decision. Determination will soon grow; fear of plunging into life will disappear, and the experiences gained will guide our mind to better judgment.

To eradicate Ignorance, again let us not be afraid of experience, but with mind awake and with eyes and ears wide open take in every particle of knowledge which may be obtained. At the same time we must keep flexible in thought, lest preconceived ideas and former convictions rob us of the opportunity of gaining fresh and wider knowledge. We should be ever ready to expand the mind and to disregard any idea, however firmly rooted, if under wider experience a greater truth shows itself.

Like Pride, Greed is a great obstacle to advancement, and both of these must be ruthlessly washed away. The results of Greed are serious indeed, because it leads us to interfere with the soul-development of our fellow-men. We must realise that every being is here to develop his own evolution according to the dictates of his Soul, and his Soul alone, and that none of us must do anything but encourage our brother in that development. We must help him to hope and, if in our power, increase his knowledge and worldly opportunities to gain his advancement. Just as we would wish others to help us up the steep and difficult mountain path of life, so let us be ever ready to lend a helping hand and give the experience of our wider knowledge to a weaker or younger brother. Such should be the attitude of parent to child, master to man or comrade to comrade, giving care, love and protection as far as may be needed and beneficial, yet never for one moment interfering with the natural evolution of the personality, as this must be dictated by the Soul.

Many of us in our childhood and early life are much nearer to our own Soul than we are in later years, and have then clearer ideas of our work in life, the endeavours we are expected to make and the character we are required to develop. The reason for this is that the materialism and circumstances of our age, and the personalities with whom we associate, lead us away from the voice of our Higher Self and bind us firmly to the commonplace with its lack of ideals, all too evident in this civilisation. Let the parent, the master and the comrade ever strive to encourage the growth of the Higher Self within those over whom they have the wonderful privilege and opportunity to exert their influence, but let them ever allow freedom to others, as they hope to have freedom given to them.

So in a similar way may we seek out any faults in our constitution and wash them out by developing the opposing virtue, thus removing from our nature the cause of the conflict between Soul and personality, which is the primary basic cause of disease. Such action alone, if the patient has faith and strength, will bring relief, health and joy, and in those not so strong will materially assist the work of the earthly physician in bringing about the same result.

We must earnestly learn to develop individuality according to the dictates of our own Soul, to fear no man and to see that no one interferes with, or dissuades us from, the development of our evolution, the fulfilment of our duty and the rendering of help to our fellow-men, remembering that the further we advance, the greater blessing we become to those around. Especially must we be on guard in the giving of help to other people, no matter whom they be, to be certain that the desire to help comes from the dictates of the Inner Self and is not a false sense of duty imposed by the suggestion or persuasion of a more dominant personality. One tragedy resulting from modern convention is of such a type, and it is impossible to calculate the thousands of hindered lives, the myriads of missed opportunities, the sorrow and the suffering so caused, the countless number of children who from a sense of duty have perhaps for years waited upon an invalid when the only malady the parent has known has been the greed of attention. Think of the armies of men and women who have been prevented from doing perhaps some great and useful work for humanity because their personality has been captured by some one individual from whom they have not had the courage to win freedom; the children who in their early days know and desire their ordained calling, and yet from difficulties of circumstance, dissuasion by others and weakness of purpose glide into some other branch of life, where they are neither happy nor able to develop their evolution as they might otherwise have done. It is the dictates of our conscience alone which can tell us whether our duty lies with one or many, how and whom we should serve; but whichever it may be, we should obey that command to the utmost of our ability.

Finally, let us not fear to plunge into life; we are here to gain experience and knowledge, and we shall learn but little unless we face realities and seek to our utmost. Such experience can be gained in every quarter, and the truths of nature and of humanity can be won just as effectively, perhaps even more so, in a country cottage as amongst the noise and hustle of a city.

CHAPTER FIVE

As lack of individuality (that is, the allowing of interference with the personality, such interference preventing it from complying with the demands of the Higher Self) is of such great importance in the production of disease, and as it often begins early in life, let us now consider the true relation between parent and child, teacher and pupil.

Fundamentally, the office of parenthood is to be the privileged means (and, indeed, it should be considered as divinely privileged) of enabling a soul to contact this world for the sake of evolution. If properly understood, there is probably no greater opportunity offered to mankind than this, to be the agent of the physical birth of a soul and to have the care of the young personality during the first few years of its existence on earth. The whole attitude of parents should be to give the little newcomer all the spiritual, mental and physical guidance to the utmost of their ability, ever remembering that the wee one is an individual soul come down to gain his own experience and knowledge in his own way according to the dictates of his Higher Self, and every possible freedom should be given for unhampered development.

The office of parenthood is one of divine service, and should be respected as much as, or perhaps even more than, any other duty we may be called upon to undertake. As it is one of sacrifice, it must ever be borne in mind that nothing whatever should be required in return from the child, the whole object being to give, and give alone, gentle love, protection and guidance until the soul takes charge of the young personality. Independence, individuality and freedom, should be taught from the beginning, and the child should be encouraged as early as possible in life to think and act for himself. All parental control should be relinquished step by step as the ability for self-management is developed, and later on no restraint or false idea of duty to parenthood should hamper the dictates of the child's soul.

Parenthood is an office in life which passes from one to another, and is in essence a temporary giving of guidance and protection for a brief period, after which time it should then cease its efforts and leave the object of its attention free to advance alone. Be it remembered that the child for whom we may become a temporary guardian may be a much older and greater soul than ourselves, and spiritually our superior, so that control and protection should be confined to the needs of the young personality.

Parenthood is a sacred duty, temporary in its character and passing from generation to generation. It carries with it nothing but service and calls for no obligation in return from the young, since they must be left free to develop in their own way and become as fitted as possible to fulfil the same office in but a few years' time. Thus the child should have no restrictions, no obligations and no parental hindrances, knowing that parenthood had previously been bestowed on his father and mother and that it may be his duty to perform the same office for another.

Parents should be particularly on guard against any desire to mould the young personality according to their own ideas or wishes, and should refrain from any undue control or demand of favours in return for their natural duty and divine privilege of being the means of helping a soul to contact the world. Any desire for control, or wish to shape the young life for personal motives, is a terrible form of greed and should never be countenanced, for if in the young father or mother this takes root it will in later years lead them to be veritable vampires. If there is the least desire to dominate, it should be checked at the onset. We must refuse to be under the slavery of greed, which compels in us the wish to possess others. We must encourage in ourselves the art of giving, and develop this until it has washed out by its sacrifice every trace of adverse action.

The teacher should ever bear in mind that it is his office merely to be the agent of giving to the young guidance and an opportunity of learning the things of the world and of life, so that each child may absorb knowledge in his own way, and, if allowed freedom, instinctively choose that which is necessary for the success of his life. Again, therefore, nothing more than the gentlest care and guidance should be given to enable the student to gain the knowledge he requires.

Children should remember that the office of parenthood, as emblematical of creative power, is divine in its mission, but that it calls for no restriction of development and no obligations which might hamper the life and work dictated to them by their own Soul. It is impossible to estimate in this present civilisation the untold suffering, the cramping of natures and the developing of dominant characters which the lack of a realisation of this fact produces. In almost every home parents and children build themselves prisons from entirely false motives and a wrong conception of the relationship of parent and child. These prisons bar the freedom, cramp the life, prevent the natural development and bring unhappiness to all concerned, and the mental, nervous and even physical disorders which afflict such people form a very large proportion indeed of the sickness of our present time.

It cannot be too firmly realised that every soul in incarnation is down here for the specific purpose of gaining experience and understanding, and of perfecting his personality towards those ideals laid down by the soul. No matter what our relationship be to each other, whether husband and wife, parent and child, brother and sister, or master and man, we sin against our Creator and against our fellow-men if we hinder from motives of personal desire the evolution of another soul. Our sole duty is to obey the dictates of our own conscience, and this will never for one moment brook the domination of another personality. Let everyone remember that his Soul has laid down for him a particular work, and that unless he does this work, though perhaps not consciously, he will inevitably raise a conflict between his Soul and personality which of necessity reacts in the form of physical disorders.

True, it may be the calling of any one individual to devote his life to one other alone, but before doing so let him be absolutely certain that this is the command of his Soul, and that it is not the suggestion of some other dominant personality over-persuading him, or false ideas of duty misdirecting him. Let him also remember that we come down into this world to win battles, to gain strength against those who would control us, and to advance to that stage when we pass through life doing our duty quietly and calmly, undeterred and uninfluenced by any living being, calmly guided always by the voice of our Higher Self. For very many their greatest battle will be in their own home, where before gaining their liberty to win victories in the world they will have to free themselves from the adverse domination and control of some very near relative.

Any individual, whether adult or child, part of whose work it is in this life to free himself from the dominant control of another, should remember the following: firstly, that his would-be oppressor should be regarded in the same way as we look upon an opponent in sport, as a personality with whom we are playing the game of Life, without the least trace of bitterness, and that if it were not for such opponents we should be lacking the opportunity of developing our own courage and individuality; secondly, that the real victories of life come through love and gentleness, and that in such a contest no force whatever must be used: that by steadily growing in his own nature, bearing sympathy, kindness and, if possible, affection – or, even better, love – towards the opponent, he may so develop that in time he may very gently and quietly follow the call of conscience without allowing the least interference.

Those who are dominant require much help and guidance to enable them to realise the great universal truth of Unity and to understand the joy of Brotherhood. To miss such things is to miss the real happiness of Life, and we must help such folk as far as lies within our power. Weakness on our part, which allows them to extend their influence, will in no way assist them; a gentle refusal to be under their control and an endeavour to bring to them the realisation of the joy of giving will help them along the upward path.

The gaining of our freedom, the winning of our individuality and independence, will in most cases call for much courage and faith. But in the darkest hours, and when success seems well-nigh impossible, let us ever remember that God's children should never be afraid, that our Souls only give us such tasks as we are capable of accomplishing, and that with our own courage and faith in the Divinity within us victory must come to all who continue to strive.

CHAPTER SIX

And now, dear brothers and sisters, when we realise that Love and Unity are the great foundations of our Creation, that we in ourselves are children of the Divine Love, and that the eternal conquest of all wrong and suffering will be accomplished by means of gentleness and love, when we realise all this, where in this beauteous picture are we to place such practices as vivisection and animal gland grafting? Are we still so primitive, so pagan, that we yet believe that by the sacrifice of animals we are enabled to escape the results of our own faults and failings? Nearly 2,500 years ago the Lord Buddha showed to the world the wrongness of sacrificing the lower creatures. Humanity already owes a mighty debt to the animals which it has tortured and destroyed, and far from any good resulting to man from such inhuman practices, nothing but harm and damage can be wrought to both the human and animal kingdoms. How far have we of the West wandered from those beautiful ideals of our Mother India of old times, when so great was the love for the creatures of the earth that men were trained and skilled to attend the maladies and injuries of not only the animals, but also the birds. Moreover, there were vast sanctuaries for all types of life, and so averse were the people to hurting a lower creature that any man who hunted was refused the attendance of a physician in time of sickness until he had vowed to relinquish such a practice.

Let us not speak against the men who practise vivisection, for numbers of these are working with truly humanitarian principles, hoping and striving to find some relief for human suffering; their motive is good enough, but their wisdom is poor, and they have little understanding of the reason of life. Motive alone, however right, is not enough; it must be combined with wisdom and knowledge.

Of the horror of the black magic associated with gland grafting let us not even write, but implore every human being to shun it as ten thousand times worse than any plague, for it is a sin against God, man and animal.

With just such one or two exceptions there is no point in dwelling on the failure of modern medical science; destruction is useless unless we rebuild a better edifice, and as in medicine the foundation of the newer building is already laid, let us concentrate on adding one or two stones to that temple. Neither is adverse criticism of the profession to-day of value; it is the system which is mainly wrong, not the men; for it is a system whereby the physician, from economic reasons alone, has not the time for administering quiet, peaceful treatment or the opportunity for the necessary meditation and thought which should be the heritage of those who devote their lives to attendance on the sick. As Paracelsus said, the wise physician

attends five, not fifteen, patients in a day – an ideal impractic-
able in this age for the average practitioner.

The dawn of a new and better art of healing is upon us. A
hundred years ago the Homeopathy of Hahnemann was as the
first streak of the morning light after a long night of darkness,
and it may play a big part in the medicine of the future.
Moreover, the attention which is being given at the present
time to improving conditions of life and providing purer and
cleaner diet is an advance towards the prevention of sickness;
and those movements which are directed to bring to the notice
of the people both the connection between spiritual failings and
disease and the healing which may be obtained through
perfection of the mind, are pointing the way towards the
coming of that bright sunshine in whose radiant light the
darkness of disease will disappear.

Let us remember that disease is a common enemy, and that
every one of us who conquers a fragment of it is thereby
helping not only himself but the whole of humanity. A certain,
but definite, amount of energy will have to be expended before
its overthrow is complete; let us one and all strive for this
result, and those who are greater and stronger than the others
may not only do their share, but materially assist their weaker
brothers.

Obviously the first way to prevent the spread and increase of
disease is for us to cease committing those actions which
extend its power; the second, to wipe out from our natures our

own defects, which would allow further invasion. The achievement of this is victory indeed; then, having freed ourselves, we are free to help others. And it is not so difficult as it may at first appear; we are but expected to do our best, and we know that this is possible for all of us if we will but listen to the dictates of our own Soul. Life does not demand of us unthinkable sacrifice; it asks us to travel its journey with joy in our heart and to be a blessing to those around, so that if we leave the world just that trifle better for our visit, then have we done our work.

The teachings of religions, if properly read, plead with us 'to forsake all and follow Me', the interpretation of which is to give ourselves entirely up to the demands of our Higher Self, but not, as some imagine, to discard home and comfort, love and luxury; very far from this is the truth. A prince of the realm, with all the glories of the palace, may be a Godsend and a blessing indeed to his people, to his country – nay, even to the world; how much might have been lost had that prince imagined it his duty to enter a monastery. The offices of life in every branch, from the lowliest to the most exalted, have to be filled, and the Divine Guide of our destinies knows into which office to place us for our best advantage; all we are expected to do is to fulfil that duty cheerfully and well. There are saints at the factory bench and in the stokehold of a ship as well as among the dignitaries of religious orders. Not one of us upon this earth is being asked to do more than is within his power to perform, and if we strive to obtain the best within us, ever guided by our Higher Self, health and happiness is a possibility for each one.

For the greater part of the last two thousand years Western civilisation has passed through an age of intense materialism, and the realisation of the spiritual side of our natures and existence has been greatly lost in the attitude of mind which has placed worldly possessions, ambitions, desires and pleasures above the real things of life. The true reason of man's existence on earth has been overshadowed by his anxiety to obtain from his incarnation nothing but worldly gain. It has been a period when life has been very difficult because of the lack of the real comfort, encouragement and uplift which is brought by a realisation of greater things than those of the world. During the last centuries religions have to many people appeared rather as legends having no bearing on their lives instead of being the very essence of their existence. The true nature of our Higher Self, the knowledge of previous and later life, apart from this present one, has meant but very little to us instead of being the guide and stimulus of our every action. We have rather shunned the great things and attempted to make life as comfortable as possible by putting the super-physical out of our minds and depending upon earthly pleasures to compensate us for our trials. Thus have position, rank, wealth and worldly possessions become the goal of these centuries; and as all such things are transient and can only be obtained and held with much anxiety and concentration on material things, so has the real internal peace and happiness of the past generations been infinitely below that which is the due of mankind.

The real peace of the Soul and mind is with us when we are making spiritual advance, and it cannot be obtained by the accumulation of wealth alone, no matter how great. But the times are changing, and the indications are many that this civilisation has begun to pass from the age of pure materialism to a desire for the realities and truths of the universe. The general and rapidly increasing interest exhibited to-day for knowledge of superphysical truths, the growing number of those who are desiring information on existence before and after this life, the founding of methods to conquer disease by faith and spiritual means, the quest after the ancient teachings and wisdom of the East – all these are signs that people of the present time have glimpsed the reality of things. Thus, when we come to the problem of healing we can understand that this also will have to keep pace with the times and change its methods from those of gross materialism to those of a science founded upon the realities of Truth and governed by the same Divine laws which rule our very natures. Healing will pass from the domain of physical methods of treating the physical body to that of spiritual and mental healing, which, by bringing about harmony between the Soul and mind, will eradicate the very basic cause of disease, and then allow such physical means to be used as may be necessary to complete the cure of the body.

It seems quite possible that unless the medical profession realises these facts and advances with the spiritual growth of the people the art of healing may pass into the hands of religious orders or into those of the trueborn healers of men who exist in every generation, but who yet have lived more or less unobserved, prevented from following their natural calling by the attitude of the orthodox. So that the physician of the future will have two great aims. The first will be to assist the patient to a knowledge of himself and to point out to him the fundamental mistakes he may be making, the deficiencies in his character which he should remedy, and the defects in his nature which must be eradicated and replaced by the corresponding virtues. Such a physician will have to be a great student of the laws governing humanity and of human nature itself, so that he may recognise in all who come to him those elements which are causing a conflict between the Soul and the personality. He must be able to advise the sufferer how best to bring about the harmony required, what actions against Unity he must cease to perform and the necessary virtues he must develop to wipe out his defects. Each case will need a careful study, and it will only be those who have devoted much of their life to the knowledge of mankind and in whose heart burns the desire to help, who will be able to undertake successfully this glorious and divine work for humanity, to open the eyes of a sufferer and enlighten him on the reason of his being, and to inspire hope, comfort and faith which will enable him to conquer his malady.

The second duty of the physician will be to administer such remedies as will help the physical body to gain strength and assist the mind to become calm, widen its outlook and strive towards perfection, thus bringing peace and harmony to the whole personality. Such remedies there are in nature, placed there by the mercy of the Divine Creator for the healing and comfort of mankind. A few of these are known, and more are being sought at the present time by physicians in different parts of the world, especially in our Mother India, and there is no doubt that when such researches have become more developed we shall regain much of the knowledge which was known more than two thousand years ago, and the healer of the future will have at his disposal the wonderful and natural remedies which were divinely placed for man to relieve his sickness.

Thus the abolition of disease will depend upon humanity realising the truth of the unalterable laws of our Universe and adapting itself with humility and obedience to those laws, thus bringing peace between its Soul and itself, and gaining the real joy and happiness of life. And the part of the physician will be to assist any sufferer to a knowledge of such truth and to point out to him the means by which he can gain harmony, to inspire him with faith in his Divinity which can

overcome all, and to administer such physical remedies as will
help in the harmonising of the personality and the healing of
the body.

CHAPTER SEVEN

And now we come to the all-important problem, how can we help ourselves? How can we keep our mind and body in that state of harmony which will make it difficult or impossible for disease to attack us, for it is certain that the personality without conflict is immune from illness.

First let us consider the mind. We have already discussed at some length the necessity of seeking within ourselves those defects we possess which cause us to work against Unity and out of harmony with the dictates of the Soul, and of eliminating these faults by developing the opposing virtues. This can be done on the lines already indicated, and an honest self-examination will disclose to us the nature of our errors. Our spiritual advisers, true physicians and intimate friends should all be able to assist us to obtain a faithful picture of ourselves, but the perfect method of learning this is by calm thought and meditation, and by bringing ourselves to such an atmosphere of peace that our Souls are able to speak to us through our conscience and intuition, and to guide us according to their wishes. If we can only set aside a short time every day, quite alone and in as quiet a place as possible, free from interruption, and merely sit or lie quietly, either keeping the mind a blank or calmly thinking of one's work in life, it will be found after a time that we get great help at such moments and, as it were, flashes of knowledge and guidance are given to us. We find that the questions of the difficult problems of life are unmistakably answered, and we become able to choose with confidence the right course. Throughout such times we should keep an earnest desire in the heart to serve humanity and work according to the dictates of our Soul.

Be it remembered that when the fault is found the remedy lies not in a battle against this and not in a use of will power and energy to suppress a wrong, but in a steady development of the opposite virtue, thus automatically washing from our natures all trace of the offender. This is the true and natural method of advancement and of the conquest of wrong, vastly easier and more effective than fighting a particular defect. To struggle against a fault increases its power, keeps our attention riveted on its presence, and brings us a battle indeed, and the most success we can then expect is conquest by suppression, which is far from satisfactory, as the enemy is still with us and may in a weak moment show itself afresh. To forget the failing and consciously to strive to develop the virtue which would make the former impossible, this is true victory.

For example, should there be cruelty in our nature, we can continually say, 'I will not be cruel', and so prevent ourselves erring in that direction; but the success of this depends on the strength of the mind, and should it weaken we might for the moment forget our good resolve. But should we, on the other hand, develop real sympathy towards our fellow-men, this quality will once and for all make cruelty impossible, for we should shun the very act with horror because of our fellow-feeling. About this there is no suppression, no hidden enemy to come forward at moments when we are off our guard, because our sympathy will have completely eradicated from our nature the possibility of any act which could hurt another.

As we have previously seen, the nature of our physical maladies will materially help in pointing out to us the mental disharmony which is the basic cause of their origin; and another great factor of success is that we must have a zest for life and look upon existence not merely as a duty to be borne with as much patience as possible, developing a real joy in the adventure of our journey through this world.

Perhaps one of the greatest tragedies of materialism is the development of boredom and the loss of real inner happiness; it teaches people to seek contentment and compensation for troubles in earthly enjoyments and pleasures, and these can never bring anything but temporary oblivion of our difficulties. Once we begin to seek compensation for our trials at the hands of the paid jester we start a vicious circle. Amusement, entertainment and frivolity are good for us all, but not when we persistently depend upon these to alleviate our troubles. Worldly amusements of every kind have to be steadily increased in their intensity to keep their hold, and the thrill of yesterday becomes the bore of to-morrow. So we go on seeking other and greater excitements until we become satiated and can no longer obtain relief in that direction. In some form or another rehance on worldly entertainment makes Fausts of us all, and though perhaps we may not fully realise it in our conscious self, life becomes for us little more than a patient duty and all its true zest and joy, such as should be the heritage of every child and be maintained until our latest hours, departs from us. The extreme stage is reached to-day in the scientific efforts being evolved to obtain rejuvenation, prolongation of natural life and increase of sensual pleasures by means of devilish practices.

The state of boredom is responsible for the admittance into ourselves of much more disease than would be generally realised, and as it tends to-day to occur early in life, so the maladies associated with it tend to appear at a younger age. Such a condition cannot occur if we acknowledge the truth of our Divinity, our mission in the world, and thereby possess the joy of gaining experience and helping others. The antidote for boredom is to take an active and lively interest in all around us, to study life throughout the whole day, to learn and learn and learn from our fellow-men and from the occurrences in life the Truth that lies behind all things, to lose ourselves in the art of gaining knowledge and experience, and to watch for opportunities when we may use such to the advantage of a fellow-traveller. Thus every moment of our work and play will bring with it a zeal for learning, a desire to experience real things, real adventures and deeds worth while, and as we develop this faculty we shall find that we are regaining the power of obtaining joy from the smallest incidents, and occurrences we have previously regarded as commonplace and of dull monotony will become the opportunity for research and adventure. It is in the simple things of life – the simple things because they are nearer the great Truth – that real pleasure is to be found.

Resignation, which makes one become merely an unobservant passenger on the journey of life, opens the door to untold adverse influences which would never have an opportunity of gaining admittance as long as our daily existence brought with it the spirit and joy of adventure. Whatever may be our station, whether a worker in the city with its teeming myriads or a lonely shepherd on the hills, let us strive to turn monotony into interest, dull duty into a joyous opportunity for experience, and daily life into an intense study of humanity and the great fundamental laws of the Universe. In every place there is ample opportunity to observe the laws of Creation, either in the mountains or valleys or amongst our brother men. First let us turn life into an adventure of absorbing interest, when boredom will be no longer possible, and from the knowledge thus gained seek to harmonise our mind with our Soul and with the great Unity of God's Creation.

Another fundamental help to us is to put away all fear. Fear in reality holds no place in the natural human kingdom, since the Divinity within us, which is ourself, is unconquerable and immortal, and if we could but realise it we, as Children of God, have nothing of which to be afraid. In materialistic ages fear naturally increases in earthly possessions (whether they be of the body itself or external riches), for if such things be our world, since they are so transient, so difficult to obtain and so impossible to hold save for a brief spell, they arouse in us the utmost anxiety lest we miss an opportunity of grasping them while we may, and we must of necessity live in a constant state of fear, conscious or subconscious, because in our inner self we know that such possessions may at any moment be snatched from us and that at the most we can only hold them for a brief life.

In this age the fear of disease has developed until it has become a great power for harm, because it opens the door to those things we dread and makes it easier for their admission. Such fear is really self-interest, for when we are earnestly absorbed in the welfare of others there is no time to be apprehensive of personal maladies. Fear at the present time is playing a great part in intensifying disease, and modern science has increased the reign of terror by spreading abroad to the general public its discoveries, which as yet are but half-truths. The knowledge of bacteria and the various germs associated with disease has played havoc in the minds of tens of thousands of people, and by the dread aroused in them has in itself rendered them more susceptible of attack. While lower forms of life, such as bacteria, may play a part in or be associated with physical disease, they constitute by no means the whole truth of the problem, as can be demonstrated scientifically or by everyday occurrences. There is a factor which science is unable to explain on physical grounds, and that is why some people become affected by disease whilst others escape, although both classes may be open to the same possibility of infection. Materialism forgets that there is a factor above the physical plane which in the ordinary course of life protects or renders susceptible any particular individual with regard to disease, of whatever nature it may be. Fear, by its depressing effect on our mentality, thus causing disharmony in our physical and magnetic bodies, paves the way for invasion, and if bacteria and such physical means were the sure and only cause of disease, then indeed there might be but little encouragement not to be afraid. But when we realise that in the worst epidemics only a proportion of those exposed to infection are attacked and that, as we have already seen, the real cause of disease lies in our own personality and is within our control, then have we reason to go about without dread and fearless, knowing that the remedy lies with ourselves. We can put all fear of physical means alone as a cause of disease out of our minds, knowing that such anxiety merely renders us susceptible, and that if we are endeavouring to bring harmony into our personality we need anticipate illness no more than we dread being struck by lightning or hit by a fragment of a falling meteor.

Now let us consider the physical body. It must never be forgotten that this is but the earthly habitation of the Soul, in which we dwell only for a short time in order that we may be able to contact the world for the purpose of gaining experience and knowledge. Without too much identifying ourselves with our bodies we should treat them with respect and care, so that they may be healthy and last the longer to do our work. Never for one moment should we become engrossed or over-anxious about them, but learn to be as little conscious of their existence as possible, using them as a vehicle of our Soul and mind and as servants to do our will. External and internal cleanliness are of great importance. For the former we of the West use our water too hot; this opens the skin and allows the admission of dirt. Moreover, the excessive use of soap renders the surface sticky. Cool or tepid water, either running as a shower bath or changed more than once is nearer the natural method and keeps the body healthier; only such an amount of soap as is necessary to remove obvious dirt should be used, and this should afterwards be well washed off in fresh water.

Internal cleanliness depends on diet, and we should choose everything that is clean and wholesome and as fresh as possible, chiefly natural fruits, vegetables and nuts. Animal flesh should certainly be avoided; first, because it gives rise to much physical poison in the body; secondly, because it stimulates an abnormal and excessive appetite; and thirdly, because it necessitates cruelty to the animal world. Plenty of fluid should be taken to cleanse the body, such as water and natural wines and products made direct from Nature's storehouse, avoiding the more artificial beverages of distillation.

Sleep should not be excessive, as many of us have more

control over ourselves whilst awake than when asleep. The old saying, 'Time to turn over, time to turn out', is an excellent guide as to when to rise.

Clothing should be as light in weight as is compatible with warmth; it should allow air to reach the body, and sunshine and fresh air should be permitted to contact the skin on all possible occasions. Water and sun bathing are great donors of health and vitality.

In all things cheerfulness should be encouraged, and we should refuse to be oppressed by doubt and depression, but remember that such are not of ourselves, for our Souls know only joy and happiness.

CHAPTER EIGHT

Thus we see that our conquest of disease will mainly depend on the following: Firstly, the realisation of the Divinity within our nature and our consequent power to overcome all that is wrong: secondly, the knowledge that the basic cause of disease is due to disharmony between the personality and the Soul; thirdly, our willingness and ability to discover the fault which is causing such a conflict; and fourthly, the removal of any such fault by developing the opposing virtue.

The duty of the healing art will be to assist us to the necessary knowledge and means by which we may overcome our maladies, and in addition to this to administer such remedies as will strengthen our mental and physical bodies and give us greater opportunities of victory. Then shall we indeed be capable of attacking disease at its very base with real hope of success. The medical school of the future will not particularly interest itself in the ultimate results and products of disease, nor will it pay so much attention to actual physical lesions, or administer drugs and chemicals merely for the sake of palliating our symptoms, but knowing the true cause of sickness and aware that the obvious physical results are merely secondary, it will concentrate its efforts upon bringing about that harmony between body, mind and soul which results in the relief and cure of disease. And in such cases as are undertaken early enough the correction of the mind will avert the imminent illness.

Amongst the types of remedies that will be used will be those obtained from the most beautiful plants and herbs to be found in the pharmacy of Nature, such as have been divinely enriched with healing powers for the mind and body of man.

For our own part we must practise peace, harmony, individuality and firmness of purpose and increasingly develop the knowledge that in essence we are of Divine origin, children of the Creator, and thus have within us, if we will but develop it, as in time we ultimately surely must, the power to attain perfection. And this reality must increase within us until it becomes the most outstanding feature of our existence. We must steadfastly practise peace, imagining our minds as a lake ever to be kept calm, without waves, or even ripples, to disturb its tranquillity, and gradually develop this state of peace until no event of life, no circumstance, no other personality is able under any condition to ruffle the surface of that lake or raise within us any feelings of irritability, depression or doubt. It will materially help to set apart a short time each day to think quietly of the beauty of peace and the benefits of calmness, and to realise that it is neither by worrying nor hurrying that we accomplish most, but by calm, quiet thought and action become more efficient in all we undertake. To harmonise our conduct in this life in accordance with the wishes of our own

Soul, and to remain in such a state of peace that the trials and disturbances of the world leave us unruffled, is a great attainment indeed and brings to us that Peace which passeth understanding; and though at first it may seem to be beyond our dreams, it is in reality, with patience and perseverance, within the reach of us all.

We are not all asked to be saints or martyrs or men of renown; to most of us less conspicuous offices are allotted. But we are all expected to understand the joy and adventures of life and to fulfil with cheerfulness the particular piece of work which has been ordained for us by our Divinity.

For those who are sick, peace of mind and harmony with the Soul is the greatest aid to recovery. The medicine and nursing of the future will pay much more attention to the development of this within the patient than we do to-day when, unable to judge the progress of a case except by materialistic scientific means, we think more of the frequent taking of temperature and a number of attentions which interrupt, rather than promote, that quiet rest and relaxation of body and mind which are so essential to recovery. There is no doubt that at the very onset of, at any rate, minor ailments, if we could but get a few hours' complete relaxation and in harmony with our Higher Self the illness would be aborted. At such moments we need to bring down into ourselves but a fraction of that calm, as symbolised by the entry of Christ into the boat during the storm on the lake of Galilee, when He ordered 'Peace, be still'.

Our outlook on life depends on the nearness of the personality to the Soul. The closer the union the greater the harmony and peace, and the more clearly will shine the light of Truth and the radiant happiness which is of the higher realms; these will hold us steady and undismayed by the difficulties and terrors of the world, since they have their foundations on the Eternal Truth of Good. The knowledge of Truth also gives to us the certainty that, however tragic some of the events of the world may appear to be, they form but a temporary stage in the evolution of man; and that even disease is in itself beneficent and works under the operation of certain laws designed to produce ultimate good and exerting a continual pressure towards perfection. Those who have this knowledge are unable to be touched or depressed or dismayed by those events which are such a burden to others, and all uncertainty, fear and despair go for ever. If we can but keep in constant communion with our own Soul, our Heavenly Father, then indeed is the world a place of joy, nor can any adverse influence be exerted upon us.

We are not permitted to see the magnitude of our own Divinity, or to realise the mightiness of our Destiny and the glorious future which lies before us; for, if we were, life would be no trial and would involve no effort, no test of merit. Our virtue lies in being oblivious for the most part to those great things, and yet having faith and courage to live well and master the difficulties of this earth. We can, however, by communion with our Higher Self, keep that harmony which enables us to overcome all worldly opposition and make our journey along the straight path to fulfil our destiny, undeterred by the influences which would lead us astray.

Next must we develop individuality and free ourselves from all worldly influences, so that obeying only the dictates of our own Soul and unmoved by circumstances or other people we become our own masters, steering our bark over the rough seas of life without ever quitting the helm of rectitude, or at any time leaving the steering of our vessel to the hands of another. We must gain our freedom absolutely and completely, so that all we do, our every action – nay, even our every thought – derives its origin in ourselves, thus enabling us to live and give freely of our own accord, and of our own accord alone.

Our greatest difficulty in this direction may lie with those nearest to us in this age when the fear of convention and false standards of duty are so appallingly developed. But we must increase our courage, which with so many of us is sufficient to face the apparently big things of life, but which yet fails at the more intimate trials. We must be able with impersonality to determine right and wrong and to act fearlessly in the presence of relative or friend. What a vast number of us are heroes in the outer world, but cowards at home! Though subtle indeed may be the means used to prevent us from fulfilling our Destiny, the pretence of love and affection, or a false sense of duty, methods to enslave us and keep us prisoners to the wishes and desires of others, yet must all such be ruthlessly put aside. The voice of our own Soul, and that voice alone, must be heeded as regards our duty if we are not to be hampered by those around us. Individuality must be developed to the utmost, and we must learn to walk through life relying on none but our own Soul for guidance and help, to take our freedom with both hands and plunge into the world to gain every particle of knowledge and experience which may be possible.

At the same time we must be on our guard to allow to everyone their freedom also, to expect nothing from others, but, on the contrary, to be ever ready to lend a helping hand to lift them upwards in times of their need and difficulty. Thus every personality we meet in life, whether mother, husband, child, stranger or friend, becomes a fellow-traveller, and any one of them may be greater or smaller than ourselves as regards spiritual development; but all of us are members of a common brotherhood and part of a great community making the same journey and with the same glorious end in view.

We must be steadfast in the determination to win, resolute in the will to gain the mountain summit; let us not give a moment's regret to the slips by the way. No great ascent was ever made without faults and falls, and they must be regarded as experiences which will help us to stumble less in the future. No thoughts of past errors must ever depress us; they are over and finished, and the knowledge thus gained will help to avoid a repetition of them. Steadily must we press forwards and onwards, never regretting and never looking back, for the past of even one hour ago is behind us, and the glorious future with its blazing light ever before us. All fear must be cast out; it should never exist in the human mind, and is only possible when we lose sight of our Divinity. It is foreign to us because as Sons of the Creator, Sparks of the Divine Life, we are invincible, indestructible and unconquerable. Disease is apparently cruel because it is the penalty of wrong thought and wrong action, which must result in cruelty to others. Hence the necessity of developing the love and brotherhood side of our natures to the utmost, since this will make cruelty in the future an impossibility.

The development of Love brings us to the realisation of Unity, of the truth that one and all of us are of the One Great Creation.

The cause of all our troubles is self and separateness, and this vanishes as soon as Love and the knowledge of the great Unity become part of our natures. The Universe is God rendered objective; at its birth it is God reborn; at its close it is God more highly evolved. So with man; his body is himself externalised, an objective manifestation of his internal nature; he is the expression of himself, the materialisation of the qualities of his consciousness.

In our Western civilisation we have the glorious example, the great standard of perfection and the teachings of the Christ to guide us. He acts for us as Mediator between our personality and our Soul. His mission on earth was to teach us how to obtain harmony and communion with our Higher Self, with

Our Father which is in Heaven, and thereby to obtain perfection in accordance with the Will of the Great Creator of all.

Thus also taught the Lord Buddha and other great Masters who have come down from time to time upon the earth to point out to men the way to attain perfection. There is no halfway path for humanity. The Truth must be acknowledged, and man must unite himself with the infinite scheme of Love of his Creator.

And so come out, my brothers and sisters, into the glorious sunshine of the knowledge of your Divinity, and earnestly and steadfastly set to work to join in the Grand Design of being happy and communicating happiness, uniting with that great band of the White Brotherhood whose whole existence is to obey the wish of their God, and whose great joy is in the service of their younger brother men.

For general information about the work of Dr Edward Bach and to learn more, please contact:

The Dr Edward Bach Centre
Mount Vernon
Sotwell
Wallingford
Oxon OX10 0PZ
England

ALSO AVAILABLE FROM VERMILION

Bach Flower Remedies for Animals	0091906512	£10.99
Bach Flower Remedies for Women	0091906547	£6.99
Dictionary of the Bach Flower Remedies	0091906490	£4.99
Illustrated Handbook of the Bach Flower Remedies	0091906482	£12.99
The Bach Flower Remedies Step by Step	0091906539	£4.99
The Bach Remedies Workbook	0091906520	£10.99

FREE POST AND PACKING
Overseas customers allow £2.00 per paperback

ORDER:

By phone: 01624 677237

By post: Random House Books
c/o Bookpost
PO Box 29
Douglas
Isle of Man, IM99 1BQ

By fax: 01624 670923

By email: bookshop@enterprise.net

Cheques (payable to Bookpost) and credit cards accepted

The prices shown above are correct at time of going to press. However, the
publishers reserve the right to increase prices on covers from those previously
advertised, without further notice

Allow 28 days for delivery.

When placing your order, please mention if you do not wish to receive
any additional information

www.randomhouse.co.uk